REVERSING HEART DISEASE

The truth about reversing and preventing heart diseases revealed,(scientific approach)

TABLE OF CONTENTS

legal responsibility or blame be held against the publisher for any reparation, damages, or monetary loss due to the information herein, either directly or indirectly.

Respective authors own all copyrights not held by the publisher.

The information herein is offered for informational purposes solely, and is universal as so. The presentation of the information is without contract or any type of guarantee assurance.

The trademarks that are used are without any consent, and the publication of the trademark is without permission or backing by the trademark owner. All trademarks and brands within this book are for clarifying purposes only and are the owned by the owners themselves, not affiliated with this document.

INTRODUCTION

For many heart patients finding a way for reversing heart disease is a dream while for others it may be a goal, which they believe may someday be available. When many professionals talks about reversing heart disease they may be referring to the possibility of halting, or at least slowing the progression of the disease. Many cardiologists state that reversing damage done to the heart is not within the scope of today's medicine and that many surgical techniques can repair damaged blood vessels and even the heart valves, but are dubious about the use of natural medications to reverse any damage already done by heart disease.

Many heart experts claim that once a heart is broke, it is nearly impossible to fix. Valves can be replaced and vessel repaired but there is no known way to allow the body to heal on its own, as far as heart disease is concerned. Many claims of reversing heart disease focus on the effects of a person's lifestyle and diet has the future of their heart health.

For years the medical community has a drawn a direct correlation between a person's diet and heart disease. Add to that a lack of exercise and the stage is set for a heart attack. However, some medical professionals dispute the diet-heart connection as being total and point to many other ways of reversing heart disease than a vegetarian lifestyle.

Focus On Overall Individual Health.

While disputes continued over the relationship of diet and heart disease, everyone agrees that eating nutritious meals instead of nutrition-empty calories will have a beneficial effect on reversing heart disease. Exercise is also important as studies have repeatedly shown a connection between a healthy heart and a person's weight.

When a person is significantly overweight, the heart has to work harder and while under stress may simply give up, causing a heart attack. An overweight person can begin reversing heart disease by losing weight to a level that matches their height and body type. Eating healthy, balanced meals to achieve weight loss is much better for reversing heart disease than crash dieting that can starve the body of vitamins and minerals needed for health.

Lifestyle changes including eating right and exercising can go a long way towards reversing heart disease, but once the heart muscle is damaged, there is no known way to heal it on its own. Heart transplants have been successful, but replacing the heart is in no way part of reversing heart disease.

Common Vitamins and over the counter products can help with Heart Disease such as Vitamin E, Potassium andPhytosterols.

Vitamin E may have a role in reducing the risk of lung cancer, according to researchers at the Johns Hopkins School of Hygiene and Public Health. It supplies oxygen to the heart and other muscles of the body and aids in the functioning of the immune system.

Potassium may help prevent high blood pressure and protect against artherosclerosis and reduce the risk of stroke.

Phytosterols is found in flax seed and peanuts, which are suggested to help lower serum cholesterol.

CHAPTER 1

INFLAMMATION

Inflammatory heart disease is a disease in which the heart muscles become inflamed which in turn occurs due to an infection from bacteria or viruses or even from certain internal peculiarities. When such inflammation occurs, it normally also causes rheumatic fever and the inflammation is also associated with Kawasaki disease. Before proceeding further with finding out more about how to treat such form of heart disease, it does pay to find out more about its different types.

There are three main types of inflammatory heart disease. These include myocarditis and pericarditis and endocarditis. Myocarditis is an inflammation that develops within the heart muscles and is induced because of different kinds of infections. Normally, these infections are related to viruses such as sarcodiosis and also to certain immune system diseases.

Actually, myocarditis is quite an asymptomatic condition. However, it does lead to experiencing pain in the chest region and this is in fact a major symptom that you need to be alert to. When the condition turns astringent, it can cause the heart muscles to degenerate which may then cause a heart failure.

The diagnosis of this form of inflammatory heart disease involves use of ECG as well as MRI and even blood tests. The prognosis for myocarditis is that it is not clear whether the patient will recover during the initial stages of the condition. Even so, a great number of myocarditis patients do recover from the condition though others might experience heart failure that occurs because of severe damage to the heart muscles.

Pericarditis is the other type of inflammatory heart disease that one should know about. This is a disease in which the pericardium becomes inflamed. The pericardium is really a fluid sac which surrounds the heart and provides the latter with lubrication which reduces friction while the heart is performing its activities.

There are a variety of reasons why people develop pericarditis including tumors, cancer, metabolic disorders and infections caused by bacteria or viruses. The symptoms of pericarditis include feeling pain in the chest and this pain will be noticeably cutting and very intense and it will travel from the chest region to the shoulder blades and then back and onto the neck.

To diagnosis this form of inflammatory heart disease, doctors will need to first of all inspect and define whether the chest pain being felt is that of pericarditis or another heart problem. If the pain occurs because of pericarditis, it can be detected with the help of a stethoscope. A telltale sign is that there will be some form of inflammation that the stethoscope is able to detect.

Treating pericarditis requires using anti inflammatory medications which help to bring down the inflammation. Sometimes, the doctor might even prescribe taking of narcotic pain relievers.

The third type of inflammatory heart disease, endocarditis is really a condition in which there is infection of the endocardium (inner lining of a persons heart) which leads to significant inflammation. Endocarditis normally affects those people that happen to be using artificial valves, or who suffer from congenial birth defects and also those whose hearts have been injured at some point of time in the past.

UNDERSTANDING THE BASICS OF YOUR HEART AND HEART DISEASE

Understand the basics associated with your heart and blood vessels. Here you will get an understanding of all the different types of cardiovascular disease that can be confusing. Get a basic overview of cardiovascular disease and the conditions that can affect your heart and blood vessels.

You probably hear a lot about preventing heart disease. But maybe you're not sure what heart disease is. Is it the same thing as cardiovascular disease, coronary artery disease or other heart terms you sometimes see?

With many medical terms related to the heart and blood vessels, it's no wonder you may be puzzled or confused. Here you will have a chance to brush up on some basic terms about cardiovascular disease (CVD) that can help you stay more informed. This can then help you when you're watching the news or meeting with your doctor.

The first term to know is Cardiovascular Disease or CVD. CVD is a broad term. CVD is a large collection of diseases and conditions.

If you want to be technical, CVD refers to any disorder in any of the various parts of your heart system. Your cardiovascular system consists of your heart and all the blood vessels throughout your whole body.

Cardiovascular disease has two main mechanisms:

- Diseases of the Heart (cardio)
- Diseases of the Blood Vessels (vascular)

Everything from an aneurysm to a heart attack to varicose veins are all types of CVD. You may be born with a type of CVD (congenital) or you may acquire others later on in life possibly from a lifetime of unhealthy habits, lack of exercise, smoking, and other factors.

Here's a closer look at the two mechanisms of cardiovascular disease.

- **Diseases of the Heart**

The diseases and conditions that affect the heart are in a group known as heart disease. The heart consists of a muscle that pumps blood. Arteries supply blood to the heart muscle, and the valves make sure that the blood within the heart is pumped in the right direction. Problems can occur in any of these areas.

Just like CVD, Heart Disease is a broad term.

Here are the specific types of heart disease:

**Coronary Artery Disease (CAD)

**Coronary Heart Disease (CHD)

**Cardiomyopathy

**Valvular heart disease

**Pericardial disease

**Congenital heart disease

**Heart failure (CHF)

- **Diseases of the Blood Vessels**

Blood vessels are in basic terms hollow tubes that carry blood to the organs and tissues throughout your body.

There are 4 basic types of blood vessels:

- **Arteries.**

These blood vessels carry oxygenated blood to all parts of the body

- **Veins.**

These blood vessels carry deoxygenated blood back to your heart. That is why they have a bluish cast to their color

- **Capillaries.**

These are tiny vessels that connect your arteries and veins.

- **Lymphatics.**

Fluid that leaks out of your capillaries in order to bathe your cells.

Here are some types of blood vessel disorders:

**Arteriosclerosis and atherosclerosis

**High blood pressure (HBP) or Hypertension (HTN)

**Stroke

**Aneurysm

**Peripheral Arterial Disease (PAD) and claudication

**Vasculitis

**Venous incompetence

**Venous thrombosis or blood clot

**Varicose veins

**Lymphedema

Heart Disease is a serious condition. Watch your fatty food intake, smoking, as well as your sweet tooth intake. Both can cause serious heart problems.

It is best to start out slow when changing your diet. Eating fresh fruits and vegetables is a great way to start.

ENDOTHELIUM IMPORTANCE

One of the precursors to atherosclerosis and heart disease is endothelial dysfunction. Because endothelial dysfunction can appear years before more serious heart disease symptoms, it is wise to try and repair this problem before it turns into something more serious. It is estimated that endothelial dysfunction affects approximately 50% of those over the age of 40.

The endothelium is the cells that line the inner surface of all blood vessels including arteries and veins. Any time the endothelium fails to function as it should, this can be considered endothelial dysfunction. When the endothelium is functioning properly, it is responsible for mediation of coagulation, platelet adhesion, immune function, and control of volume and electrolyte content of the intravascular and extra vascular spaces.

Several things can cause endothelial dysfunction, including cigarette smoking and diseases like high blood pressure and diabetes. When the endothelium does not function properly, veins and arteries have difficulty dilating properly. These problems are thought to be the precursor to atherosclerosis, which is a leading cause of heart disease. However, it is possible to reverse endothelial dysfunction by paying attention to your lifestyle. Reversing endothelial dysfunction before it becomes more serious is important to protecting your cardiovascular health.

There are several changes you can make to help reverse endothelial dysfunction. Here are some suggestions to help get your body headed on the right track.

First, watch your diet. It is believed that trans fats in particular can lead to endothelial dysfunction. So, it's important to remove trans fats from your diet entirely. Read product labels looking for the words hydrogenated or partially hydrogenated. If you see these words in the ingredients, stay away.

Reduce your level of other saturated fats, too. This means reducing the amount of red meat and egg yolks you consume; making the bulk of your protein come from fish, poultry and low fat dairy products.

Another important factor in reducing endothelial dysfunction is controlling your weight. Eat right and get regular exercise to ensure that your weight falls within a normal range.

If you have high blood pressure and high cholesterol, you should treat these in order to protect endothelial function. Exercise and proper diet can help lower blood pressure and cholesterol. However, if diet and exercise don't prove to be enough, your doctor may prescribe medication to help get these numbers under control.

Another important way you can improve your endothelial function is by making sure your diet is rich in anti-oxidants. Anti-oxidants are responsible for combating free radicals in our bodies. Free radicals are created as we process our food each day. If we don't consume anti-oxidants, these free radicals can damage our DNA and cells, including the cells that make up the endothelium.

So, in addition to making sure that your diet is low in saturated and trans fats, make sure it's rich in anti-oxidant powerhouses. All fresh fruits and vegetables contain anti-oxidants, but some are more potent than others. Artichokes, asparagus, tomatoes and red beans are the best vegetables to eat and the best fruits include blueberries and pomegranates.

In addition to fruits and vegetables, anti-oxidants can be found in dark chocolate, coffee and green tea. Green tea is a particularly effective because it contains EGCG, one of the most potent anti-oxidants, belonging to the flavonol-3 class of flavonoids.

In recent years, much research has been performed on how our bodies use these flavonoids to combat free radicals and protect us from disease. This research has concluded that there are factors that determine how efficiently our bodies use the anti-oxidants we consume.

The first of these factors is our metabolism. In some situations, anti-oxidants may not be metabolized as efficiently as others. Factors that affect metabolism of anti-oxidants include our body's overall ability to process the foods we eat, including the efficiency of our digestive systems.

For example, a diet that is loaded with processed foods can cause the digestive system to slow down and may result in important nutrients being swept from the body before being absorbed properly. However, if you're eating a heart healthy diet, you'll avoid processed foods and most of this problem should be eliminated.

In addition, damaged cells appear to have more difficulty metabolizing anti-oxidants, particularly flavonoids. For this reason, if you have a significant amount of endothelial dysfunction, your body may not process the beneficial flavonoids as efficiently as we'd like.

According to a study reported by the UK Tea Council, your body's ability to metabolize the flavonoids in green tea affects the amount of benefit you'll gain in terms of restoring endothelial function. If your body is ineffective at metabolizing the flavonoids, you'll gain less benefit per cup of tea.

Of course, it's impossible for each of us to know how effectively we metabolize anti-oxidants. But, we shouldn't lose hope. Even if our bodies don't efficiently use the flavonoids we're consuming, we can make up for the deficiency simply by increasing quantity. Most doctors recommend that we drink at least three cups of green tea each day, anyway.

As with many health concerns, all the information we're given can pile up and be confusing in the long run. But, a few things are very simple. The first is that protecting our endothelial function protects us from heart disease in the long run. The second is that, along with a healthy diet and exercise, anti-oxidant rich foods like green tea can help us accomplish this.

So what if it takes a few cups each day? It just means more tea for us to enjoy!

SILENT INFLAMMATION

Silent inflammation is the general term for the underlying cause of several important diseases including heart disease, diabetes, cancer and Alzheimer's. Certain fish oil supplements have been shown to demonstrate a beneficial effect on the symptoms of these diseases. This article discusses how some medical practitioners believe this works and recommends consulting with your doctor.

Dr. Barry Sears in his book "The Anti-Inflammation Zone" defines "Silent Inflammation" as a type of inflammation that is below the threshold of pain.

The danger of silent inflammation is that you don't know it's happening in your body though it is constantly eroding your wellness over years until finally chronic disease turns up sometimes years, even decades later.

Included in the diseases that have a silent inflammation component are: heart disease, diabetes, cancer and Alzheimer's. When you are able to control inflammation you will go a long way to minimizing (if not reversing) the symptoms of chronic disease.

Dr. Sears also says, "The true key to wellness lies in also keeping a certain group of hormones, known as eicosanoids (eye-KAH-sa-noids) within a certain zone..."

His basis for saying this is that eicosanoids control inflammation, and that is becoming recognized as the underlying cause of many, if not all, chronic disease states that now threaten to destroy our health care system.

The good news is that by reversing "silent inflammation" you will:

* Think better

* Perform better

* Look better and

* Feel better

In time, by controlling the hormones that promote silent inflammation you can also:

* Help prevent heart disease and stroke

* Help ward off cancer

* Help reverse Type 2 diabetes

* Help prevent Alzheimer's, depression, Parkingson's and attention defecit disorder

* Help reduce rheumatoid arthritis, lupus and multiple sclerocis

* Help reduce severe pain from fibromyalgia, migranes, arthritis

I found one of the most impressive statements in Dr. Sears' book to be the first sentence on Chapter 7:

"The single most important thing you can do to keep silent inflammation under control is this: take a daily supplement of high dose fish oil."

ROLE OF IMMUNE SYSTEM

The immune system is wonderful system of cells and signaling cytokines that fight infections and keep us healthy. We come in contact with billions of microorganisms every day. These include bacteria, viruses, fungi, and parasites. To protect us, we have an immune system. The immune system is a fascinating collection of infection fighting white blood cells and their partners the complement system and cytokines.

Your immune system is one of the most important systems in your body. It protects you from dozens of different diseases, and it does this by fighting off large numbers of bacteria, viruses, fungi and other pathogens that attack your body every day. Furthermore, it also works to stop the initiation of cancer.

Germs are all around us, and if we weren't protected by our immune system, we would be dead in twenty-four hours. It is a complex, sophisticated, and a well organized system, and it has to be kept in top shape if you are to be fully protected. Some of the things that affect it adversely are:

• Improper nutrition

• Stress

• Overweight

• High fat diet

• Little or no exercise

• Not enough sleep

• Smoking

• Environmental toxins

• Some drugs

The white cells in your body (also known as leukocytes) are a major part of your immune system. Most are born in the marrow of your body's long bones. Some of them migrate to the thymus gland early on where they become T-cells. (The thymus is located just above the heart in the chest.) Others remain in the bone marrow, and some of them become what are called B-cells. Together, the T and B cells are referred to as lymphocytes.

While the T-cells are in the thymus they are trained to recognize over a million different antigens, with each T-cell recognizing only one specific antigen. An antigen is a molecular recognition code that is on the surface of all cells; is can be friendly or foreign. If unfriendly, such as those on viruses, it will be attacked. In most cases, however, immune system cells have to be given permission before they can attack. This is because several friendly pathogens live and perform important functions in the body. A good example is the friendly bacteria in your colon that help digest food.

Your thymus works hard to educate billions of T-cells throughout your younger years. As you grow older, however, it begins to shrink in size, and gives you less protection. That's why older people (over about 65) are more susceptible to infections and cancer.

As T-cells mature in the thymus, they take on one of four functions. They can become:

1. Helper T-cells (T-4 cells): These cells are particularly important shortly after the infection occurs. They sound the alarm, and alert the immune system, and they oversee the immune system's response. They are usually activated after particles called macrophages detect antigens; these macrophages give off cytokines, or messengers, that tell other lymphocytes to begin the attack.

2. Suppressor T-cells (T-8 cells): Once the immune system cells are sent out to fight the antigens, they must be regulated and controlled, particularly after the invaders have been defeated. If not they can attack healthy cells of the body, which may lead to autoimmune disease. Suppressor cells shut down the response when needed.

3. Killer T-cells: These cells kill by injecting poison into the cells containing the antigen. They cannot attack these cells, however, without permission from helper T-cells.

4. Natural Killer cells (NK's): They are primitive T-cells that are free to attack antigens without permission from helper T's. Basically, they are the first line of defense. Targets for them are usually identified by macrophages.

While the war between immune system cells and antigens is going on, it's important for the immune cells to be able to communicate with one another. This is done using hormone-like messengers called cytokines. One of the most important cytokines is interferon. It is released by both T-cells and macrophages, and it guides NK killers to the appropriate targets. It is also used to stop viruses from multiplying, and is helpful in impeding the development of cancer cells.

B-Cells, Antibodies, and Complement

So far we have barely mentioned the B-cells, but they also play a critical role in the war against the antigens. In particular they manufacture antibodies that attack the antigens directly. The B-cells remain in the bone marrow where they eventually become specific for many different antigens. When they mature they move to the body's lymph nodes.

When T-4 cells see a B-cell displaying the antigen of an invader, they authorize the B-cells to produce antibodies against it. The B-cells immediately begin to grow and divide into a large number of plasma cells. These plasma cells are the factories that produce antibodies. Within a few days each B-cell divides into hundreds of plasma cells, each of which produces millions of antibodies. These antibodies then head for the antigens using the bloodstream. Large numbers lock onto the antigens and disable it.

They are assisted by what is called complement. It acts as a catalyst for the reaction between the antibodies and the antigen, and it speed up the reaction. It helps neutralize viruses and other unfriendly microbes.

Phagocytes

Two other types of cells are also important in the fight against antigens. They are the neutrophils and macrophages. Known as phagocytes, they attack and eat antigens. Both are born in bone marrow, and they mature relatively fast. Neurophils are much smaller than macrophages. They are like foot soldiers - lightly armed, but there are large numbers of them, and they are usually the first to attack the antigens. When called into battle they rush in, but can only kill and eat a few antigens (10 to 20) before they die.

Macrophages start out in the thymus as monophages. When they migrate to lymphatic tissue they grow by a factor of 4 or 5 and become macrophages. They are much larger and better trained than neutrophils and they can engulf and eat up to 100 antigens. One of their major jobs is to cut microbes up into small pieces, each displaying their antigen, signaling that they are the enemy.

CHAPTER 2

CHOLESTEROL OBSESSION

Many people are aware that high levels of cholesterol are dangerous to their health because of the increase risk of heart disease and stroke. But what is cholesterol? And is it really bad for the health?

What is cholesterol? It is a combination of fatty substances and steroid naturally produced by the body. In fact, cholesterol is in every cell of our body. It makes cell membranes less fluid and holds it together without the need for a cell wall. It basically keeps the cell in the body stable. Cholesterol is also a source of energy. The liver produces 80 percent of the cholesterol but it can also be from dietary source. It also helps in digesting fats and in vitamins absorption.

What is cholesterol doing in our body? There are good and bad cholesterol. Bad cholesterol of low density lipoprotein (LDL) is produced by our body and is also needed but high level of bad cholesterol as mentioned can cause heart disease and clog the arteries. LDL are usually found in animal meat, ice cream, eggs and butter so limit the intake of these food.

What is cholesterol which known as HDL? You may heard about this before, High density lipoprotein (HDL) is also the good one which protects you from heart disease by lowering the bad cholesterol in the body. Foods high in HDL are sea foods like salmon and tuna. Foods high in fiber like fruits and vegetables also helps raise the HDL level in the body. What is cholesterol doing in our body is really important, eating more vegetables and high fiber food and limiting red meat, eggs and sweets can definitely help lower your bad HDL.

Cholesterol is not really bad for the body; it only becomes a threat if increases beyond the normal level. The truth is what is cholesterol is an essential substance which our body needs to work properly. We won't be able to function without cholesterol. The most important is the need to maintain a proper diet and exercise to make sure the good cholesterol is in a healthy level. You should also visit your doctor regularly so that you can monitor your cholesterol level and if you might need medication or a change in your diet for your cholesterol.

What is cholesterol is basically what you take in your body. If you eat unhealthy food then you'll get bad cholesterol if you eat a balanced diet coupled with exercise you'll have higher good cholesterol. It's a good lifestyle that will ensure a good health and a good level of cholesterol.

Is it really bad?

Actually no, not all cholesterol is bad. In fact, you have to have it in order for your body to function properly. Cholesterol helps your body to create cell membranes, absorb vitamin D, create bile, and it will offer itself up for the creation of hormones. Not too shabby.

The problem is that there can be too much of a good thing. High cholesterol levels can lead to serious health complications. Some of these problems are things like; high blood pressure, strokes, heart disease, and all of these medical issues can lead to death!

Cholesterol awareness

If your cholesterol is high you probably won't know it. In fact, you could do all the right things to stay healthy and still have high cholesterol. A lot of cholesterol problems stem from genetics. What this means is you need to have your cholesterol levels checked every year as part of your annual medical checkup. And like it or not, this testing should start in your early twenties.

When you get your blood tested you will want and overall score of less than 200. A doctor will be able to tell you the breakdown between the HDL and LDL levels in that score. The general rule of thumb is your LDL to HDL should be a 3-to-1 ratio. For the LDL levels you will want to be between 100 and 130 and HDL the average is 55, but higher is better.

There are many things that you can do to keep your cholesterol levels healthy. Eating right, getting exercise, and getting regular testing will help your chances of healthy cholesterol and awareness. If you are fighting genetics then you might have to follow a stricter regimen to help keep your body healthy.

That is the basics of what is cholesterol.

ABC OF CHOLESTROL

When controlling your diabetes you need go back to basics and learn the ABC's. Your ABC's are:

A = A1C

What is it?

An A1C blood test measures the percentage of hemoglobin (the oxygen-carrying protein in your red blood cells) coated with sugar. It measures your average blood glucose (sugar) level over the past two to three months. The A1C test gives you and your health care provider a measure of your progress. Most people with diabetes should have an A1C test every three to six months; people who are meeting their treatment goals may need the test only twice a year.

This lab measures your long term blood glucose control. You should have this lab at least three times a year. The recommended value from the American Diabetes Association (ADA) is less than 7%. The American Academy of Endocrinologists (AACE) recommends an A1C of less than 6.5%.

Why is it important?

The A1C test is a good measure of how well your glucose is under control. It can also be a good tool for determining if someone with prediabetes is progressing toward or has developed type 2 diabetes. Adults over age 45 with hypertension, obesity, or a family history of diabetes also are advised to get an A1C test because they have a greater risk of developing type 2 diabetes. Finding out you have an elevated A1C is a cue to make positive changes to your lifestyle.

What do the numbers mean?

- 5.7% or lower = normal blood glucose levels
- 5.8–6.4% = elevated blood glucose levels (prediabetes)
- 6.5% or higher = diabetes

What should my numbers be?

For years, people with type 2 were told to strive for an A1C of 7 percent or less, but new research indicates that one level doesn't fit all. Based on your health status, age, and risk factors, you and your health care provider should determine an A1C goal for you.

Here are the American Diabetes Association's new general guidelines:

- Person newly diagnosed with type 2 diabetes = 7% or lower
- Person with diabetes who is not prone to hypoglycemia or problems from treatment = 6.5% or lower
- Person with a history of severe hypoglycemia, limited life expectancy, or type 2 diabetes for many years = 8% or lower

B = BLOOD PRESSURE

What is it?

Blood pressure is the force of blood flow in your blood vessels. A blood pressure test reveals two readings. The top number is the systolic blood pressure, which measures the pressure as your heart beats and pushes blood through your blood vessels. The bottom number is the diastolic blood pressure, which measures the pressure when your blood vessels relax between heartbeats. People with diabetes should have their blood pressure checked at every appointment with their care provider.

High blood pressure is a sign of hypertension. You need to have your blood pressure measured every time you visit your doctor. Hypertension increases your risk for stroke (CVA), retinopathy (blindness), nephropathy (kidney disease) and neuropathy (nerve damage). The goal is less than 120/80.

Why is it important?

When your blood pressure is too high, your heart has to work harder, raising your risk for heart attack, stroke, eye problems, and kidney disease. Treating high blood pressure with diet, lifestyle changes, and medication (if needed) is important to prevent health complications.

What do the numbers mean?

- 120/80 mmHg or lower = healthy blood pressure
- 120/80–140/80 mmHg = early high blood pressure
- 140/90 or higher mmHg = high blood pressure (hypertension)

What should my numbers be?

The American Diabetes Association recommends aiming for a blood pressure below 140/90 mmHg and to take medicine if your pressure equals or exceeds that level. Exercising regularly, limiting sodium to 1,500 mg per day, and eating sufficient amount of fruits, vegetables, and low-fat dairy foods can help you control blood pressure.

C = CHOLESTEROL

What is it?

Cholesterol is a waxy, fatlike substance found in every cell in your body. It's a necessary component to produce hormones, cell membranes, and vitamin D, and to help your body digest fat. Cholesterol is also in foods that have animal origins, such as meat, poultry, seafood, and full-fat dairy products.

There are several types of cholesterol, two of which are important for people with diabetes to monitor. Low-density lipoproteins (LDL) are considered bad cholesterol and can lead to the buildup of plaque in blood vessel walls, which can cause heart attack or stroke. High-density lipoproteins (HDL) are considered good cholesterol and appear to protect against heart disease.

Triglycerides are a form of fat made in the body. People who are overweight or obese, are physically inactive, smoke, or consume large amounts of alcohol or carbohydrate are more likely to have elevated levels of triglycerides, which increases risk for heart disease.

A fasting blood test to assess your lipid profile—which measures total cholesterol, LDL and HDL cholesterol, and triglyceride levels—should be done once a year. Eating more fruits and vegetables as well as fiber-filled whole grains, exercising regularly, losing weight if necessary, and maintaining good blood glucose control can help improve your cholesterol and triglyceride levels.

High cholesterol increases your chance for a heart attack or stroke because it clogs your arteries. You should test your cholesterol at least once a year. Your goal should be to get your LDL cholesterol (lousy) cholesterol to less than 100mg/dl and your HDL cholesterol (healthy) cholesterol to greater than 50mg/dl. Also, your triglycerides (TG) should be less than 150mg/dl.

What should my numbers be?

It's important to know your cholesterol numbers and keep them in check. Your doctor will determine how often you should have your cholesterol levels tested and the numbers you should aim for.

According to the American Diabetes Association, these are the LDL, HDL, and triglycerides levels most people with diabetes should aim for:

- LDL cholesterol: Lower than 100 mg/dl
- HDL cholesterol: Higher than 40 mg/dl for men and 50 mg/dl for women is good, but HDL of 50 mg/dl or higher helps everyone lower risk for heart disease.
- Triglycerides: Lower than 150 mg/dl

How do you improve your ABCs'? Frequent monitoring of your blood glucose along with counting carbohydrates and taking your diabetic medications properly should improve your A1C. If you lose weight, stop smoking, exercise, reduce stress in your life and eat less salt and fat, you should improve your blood pressure and cholesterol levels. In addition, some people will need medications to improve their blood pressure and cholesterol. People with diabetes have a higher chance of having a heart attack or stroke than the rest of the population so improving your blood pressure and cholesterol is important.

CHOLESTROL KILLER REPUTATION

A belief need have no basis in fact. So long as the belief is confined to the believer, and helps, or at least does no harm to anyone else, then there is no problem. But this is often not the case.

Whether the belief is that you can get out of debt by taking on more debt, or that the price of a house can only rise, or that we must keep out of the sun, or that carbon dioxide is a deadly poison; beliefs have consequences. And they may do tremendous damage before they are discovered to be false or the real agenda is exposed.

There are always those that understand reality and warn of the consequences, but of course they are not listened to. If the belief is combined with money and power interests, the dissenters will be marginalised, denigrated, and may have their reputations and careers ruined.

Any professional person hates to feel helpless in the field in which they work. Doctors are a class of professional that often find themselves in that position. So when a scientist has a belief that cholesterol is bad; that reducing it provides the answer to a major killer, does it really matter if he distorts the data to 'prove' his point? He 'knows' he is right and that many lives will be saved if he can just persuade his colleagues and spread the word.

And when the rest of the medical profession hear this, a great wave of optimism is unleashed. They can now offer a solution to a terrible problem. Other scientists are enthused to carry out studies to confirm this.

These studies are criticised for their poor quality. In many cases the studies' positive conclusions are the opposite to what they actually demonstrated, but this is brushed aside. How dare you take our dream away.

A huge money flow is stimulated, making researchers very happy, making medical journals happy, providing increased prosperity for doctors, and boosting the profits of the food industry as they switch from low profit animal foods to high profit laboratory foods.

And then the drug companies come along to offer an easy solution and earn themselves a fortune in the process. And the media are very happy from all the advertising revenue flowing their way. And the public are so happy to pay for all this because they are protected from a nasty disease.

But there is a problem with all this. Cholesterol is not the villain. By focusing in the wrong area, alternative solutions - solutions that could genuinely save lives - are not considered. People are put on diets that make them miserable or make them fat, or make them unhealthy in other ways. The new dietary regime has the opposite effect. It makes people sick and they die prematurely.

And the new class of drugs cause muscle problems and liver damage and renal failure and heart failure and mental disturbances and violence and suicide and memory loss and impotency and cancer.

And it all stemmed from a belief.

The public imagine that medical research represents the highest order of precision. The reality is something quite different. It is often imprecise and carried out by people who are not trained in the scientific method. This leads to poorly designed studies containing data that are not analysed or interpreted properly. Bias is almost routine, with data twisted to fit preconceived hypothesis. To quote Dr Russell Smith: "Much of the literature therefore is nothing less than an affront to the discipline of science."

Having looked at the research into cholesterol that began in the 1950s, it is hard to disagree with physician and scientist George Mann, who described the cholesterol campaign as "the greatest scientific deception of this century, perhaps of any century."

CHAPTER 3

RISK FACTORS

Everyone needs to know what are the risk factors for heart disease because it is important. Several risk factors have to do with the foods you eat and your diet. Other factors may be things such as exercise and your cholesterol levels. Making it a point to avoid certain risks will ensure a healthier and probably longer life.

If you do not know the risk factors that are known to lead to heart disease then you could very well be endangering your own life. Practicing a heart healthy lifestyle is very important to the longevity of your life as well as others. It is also recommended that if you learn these ways early in your life you are more likely to adopt that type of lifestyle to your life, the life of your child and the life of those around you.

Your daily diet has to be the biggest factor that heavily contributes to heart disease, obesity, heart attacks and as well as many others. If your diet avoids saturated fats, processed foods, and large amounts of sugar then you should have no worries about your diet being a risk factor for heart disease.

Exercising is important in every life and should be practiced regularly. If you do not have enough physical activities in your daily life then you have a higher risk of succumbing to this type of disease as well as many other types of issues with the body and the heart.

It is always recommended to see a medical professional once a year for a routine check up on your health. At some point in time you should find out if you personally should be concerned with having high cholesterol. Your doctor will probably review your weight, height, amount of daily exercise you get as well as review what type of foods you typically eat.

The seriousness of this disease can be seen in the fact that over 40% of all people in the United States who suffer a heart attack will die from its affects.

Heart disease, which is a term that includes several more specific heart conditions, is the leading cause of death in the United States and is a major cause of disability. The major forms of this most deadly of diseases include acute rheumatic fever, chronic rheumatic heart disease, hypertensive heart disease, coronary heart disease, pulmonary heart disease, congestive heart failure and any other heart condition or disease.

It is, in simplistic terms, the inability of the heart to pump or receive adequate amounts of blood due to atherosclerosis or damage to the heart caused by infection or congenital defects. In fact heart disease and stroke both have the same risk factors and causes.

An estimated 25% of all Americans have one or more risk factors for heart disease, increasing their risk for heart attack. Most risk factors are related to lifestyle while other risk factors that cannot be changed include age, gender, and genetics.

Health behaviors associated with a high risk of heart disease include being physically inactive, eating a diet high in salt and saturated fat, and smoking tobacco. While you can't control your age, gender, race, or family history, you can decrease your chances of developing heart disease by focusing on the lifestyle changes you can make to improve your overall health.

Leading a healthy lifestyle and following medical advice to reduce or remove risk factors is the best way to reduce the risk of developing heart disease. Although heart disease takes on different specific forms, there are a common core of risk factors that influence whether someone will ultimately be at risk for heart disease or not.

There are many factors that can increase your risk of getting heart disease. Some of these factors are out of your control but most of them can be avoided by choosing to live a healthy lifestyle. Excess body fat is one of the greatest risk factors for heart disease. Cholesterol levels are determined by a combination of age, gender, heredity, and dietary choices, and of these four factors, changing your diet to a healthier one is something you can do something about. High blood pressure combined with other risk factors such as being physically inactive, eating a diet high in salt and saturated fat, and smoking tobacco greatly increases your chances of getting heart disease as well. In some cases other factors such as stress and drinking too much alcohol have been linked to cardiovascular disease.

Fortunately, many risk factors for heart disease are caused in part by unhealthy lifestyle habits, which can be altered so as to reduce one's chances of developing heart disease.

Having a blood test to determine your cholesterol levels will most likely be done and your doctor will advise you from there. High cholesterol levels are well known for being the most common risk factor of this type of disease.

Learning what are the risk factors for heart disease is the first step in preventing the actual disease from affecting you. Educating yourself about things such as getting regular exercise and eating healthy will greatly decrease your probability of having a disease of the heart. The only thing better than educating yourself, is actually practicing and committing to living a healthier life.

HIGH INSULIN

Insulin is responsible for opening up the doors to your cells so that glucose can enter. When you eat carbohydrate foods, for example rice or pasta, they are broken down into the glucose that enters your blood stream ready to be used by your cells for the purpose of providing you with energy. Once you have an excess amount of fat around your abdominal area, this process no longer works in an efficient manner.

This fat actually gets in the way of insulin function and a condition known as insulin resistance results. This means sugar will find it more and more difficult to enter your cells, even though your pancreas is producing larger amounts of insulin in the hope of moving this sugar. When this happens your body conserves it's energy source and goes into fat storage mode.

So insulin resistance brings about obesity and obesity brings about insulin resistance ... a vicious cycle! Now you have high blood sugar levels and high insulin levels ... and these high insulin levels are actually damaging your body.

Insulin is a necessary hormone for life ... in normal amounts. When your levels are four to five times higher than normal, which is the situation after your have eaten processed food, damage to your body occurs. Insulin sends a message to each and every cell, telling them to store fat and create cholesterol ... for the next eighteen hours! This is one of the reasons why people with type 2 diabetes have high cholesterol levels.

It is also one of the mechanisms that leads to people with type 2 diabetes putting on more and more weight. When you are overweight your physiology makes it even harder for you to lose weight. And again, this is one of the reasons type 2 diabetics end up with heart disease.

Many researchers have uncovered evidence that high cholesterol alone is not a risk factor for developing heart disease. But they have found, having high cholesterol levels along with type 2 diabetes, is a big risk factor for developing heart disease. In fact, studies show that just by having diabetes, the risk of heart disease is 400% higher than in non-diabetics. Even people with the metabolic syndrome, a pre-diabetic condition, are at a much higher risk as they too have high insulin levels. Their risk of developing heart disease is 300% greater compared to people without the metabolic syndrome.

Can you see how important it is to reverse your type 2 diabetes? No matter what you want to call it: a diet, an eating plan or a lifestyle plan, you are going to need to change your eating habits for the long haul!

TOXIC BLOOD AND TOXIC METALS

Toxicity has become a way life, and one that we all must cope with on a daily basis. Unfortunately we all pay a price for living in this environment. There are many factors involved as to why some individuals will pay a higher price than others.

The price we are speaking of is the impact that it has on our health. Many factors will go into determining how any individual reacts to the toxicity surrounding them. Individuals with immune systems that are at lower ebb or have been impaired for some reason or other will be more at risk to these this toxic environment. Wherever you look, be it within your own home or the great outdoors, you will be hard-pressed to find something that is not toxic to your health. Chemicals of all kinds are a way of life, and companies are coming up with more ways to include these chemicals into to our foods and products we use on a daily basis, making it very difficult, and almost impossible to avoid them. However, there are ways to avoid these pitfalls, but it will take some effort to eliminate a great many of these harmful toxic agents. The foods we eat are being processed with chemicals to preserve them and to supposedly make them more flavorful. Companies have been experimenting and finding more ways to do this. If this isn't bad enough, we cook these foods in utensils that are coated with chemicals that can possibly leech out and add toxic agents to the food we eat. We have long known that cooking in aluminum utensils can possibly cause this leeching action to occur. There is also research going on to see if this leeching out could occur in the non-stick cookware as well. As mentioned above, chemicals are everywhere, and we should be aware of the ones that can be the most detrimental to our health. We will discuss these chemicals and the affect they can have on our health.

Mercury: This has been around since Biblical times. People working the "quicksilver" mines during the times of the Pharaohs died terrible deaths at very early ages from mercury poisoning. In the early 1900's, people worked in industries that used mercury based chemicals in the manufacture of their products. The workers suffered severe muscular tremors and some even became demented. Mercury was also used in medical instruments such as the sphygmomanometer (blood pressure machine), and in the thermometers. These thermometers were used in the mouth and the possibly of breakage was always present with the possibility of mercury poisoning. These are no longer being used, and have been replaced by digital units. Mercury can also lower the T-cell counts, and known to be carcinogenic, causing cancer and other disorders such as, multiple sclerosis, and disorders of the immune system. Mercury has a tendency to affect the brain, as well as fetal tissue, resulting in brain tumors, dementia and birth defects. Mercury is found almost everywhere, in the soil, wood, rocks, oil and coal. When soil erodes it finds its way into the streams, rivers and oceans. When forests burn, mercury is released into the atmosphere. Burning coal will release mercury into the atmosphere, unless it is properly filtered. Unfortunately not enough progress has been made in this area of prevention. Mercury when it ends up in our waters will find its way into microorganisms. They in turn convert the mercury into methyl mercury. This mercury ends up in the fish that we end up eating, and then stored in our tissues.

Aluminum: A highly toxic metal found almost everywhere. It is found in many of the foods we eat because food manufacturers use it in the food emulsifiers. Also found in baking powder and some toothpaste. It is used extensively in personal deodorants, antiseptics and many of the antacids. More importantly, it is used for a great many of our cooking utensils, and this is where the leeching process will take place. Aluminum when ingested in any form, especially from the leeching process in cooking, and from all the other sources, becomes cumulative and is stored within the body. It particularly finds its way into the brain where it affects the neurons by killing them. This can cause the onset of Alzheimer's disease or dementia. Aluminum is also found in plants in the form of aluminum hydroxide. This is not like the metallic form of aluminum, and fortunately it has not been found to be harmful to the body, and that's a good thing because it is so prevalent in our environment.

Lead: Another highly toxic metal has been greatly eliminated from our environment during the last few decades. The elimination of lead based paints was one of the chief reasons for this reduction. To this day, there may be old buildings that still have the old lead based paints on their walls. The fact that lead has been decreased does not mean it has been eradicated from our environment. The immediate threat of lead today is found in our drinking water and the power plants that use coal to fuel the power needed. This burning of the coal emits clouds of vapor sending the lead into the atmosphere. Drinking water adds to our exposure to lead by as much as 20 percent. Lead is cumulative in our bodies, unless to take steps to eradicate it. Both children and adults are at risk. Children with high exposures will suffer brain damage, causing learning disabilities, behavioral problems and possible mental retardation. Damage to the nervous system is another possibility as well as ADDH. Adults can suffer numerous disorders such as, disorders of the nervous system, hypertension, forgetfulness, inability to concentrate, and pains throughout the body affecting the joints and muscles.Everyone is exposed to these metals and toxic substances and it takes considerable thought and effort to minimize exposure to them.

Do not use aluminum cooking utensils. Toxic metal can leech into the cooked foods.Do not eat fish known to have high levels of mercury. These are swordfish, albacore tuna, shark, and orange roughy.Avoid deodorants and other cosmetics that contain aluminum. There are products made of natural substances that will take the place of those with toxic additatives. Do not let a dentist put in any metal (amalgam) fillings. If you have any, a dentist experienced in the removal of amalgam fillings can replace them with the resin type. Check all household products used as laundry and dishwashing detergents. In fact check all items used for all household-cleaning chores. Check the ingredients. You will find that you can dispense with many of these products. Many will not even have all of the contained ingredients. For example, in fabric softeners, it will say, "Contains other fabric softeners". What are these other fabric softeners? Could this be "why so many people are prone to allergies and other skin disorders"? This is only the tip of the iceberg. The bottom line is, the less chemicals you use, will determine your exposure to toxic chemicals and metals.

The same holds true for all outdoor chores, gardening, etc. Gardening and lawn care can expose the individual to many toxic chemicals. There are many products that use natural ingredients to achieve the same results as those containing all the toxic chemicals. Organic gardening is the method of the future.

As previously discussed, we have all been exposed to toxic chemicals of all kinds. These have become cumulative in our bodies. Detoxifying our bodies can be a most important step in ridding our bodies of these accumulated toxic substances. An herbal detoxifier can be a way to start the detoxification process.

Research has also shown that there are two herbal items that can be a very significant method of detoxifying the body and ridding itself of heavy metals. Cilantro and Chlorella will not only help in the excretion of these metals, but can help the body to remain toxicity free.

Start the detoxification process by abstaining from eating fat and proteins so that the liver will be able start the detoxification process without putting an overload on it.

Eat only fresh vegetables and whole grains grown without pesticides, as they are the best way to detoxify the body's tissues and organs. Try to stay away from other foods except for the vegetables and whole grains, until the detoxification process has been accomplished. When this detoxification takes place, you will feel more vital and vigorous. You will have fewer headaches, muscle and joint pains, and a great deal more energy. Then, and only then, you can start adding the proteins and fats that your body requires on a daily basis. To further help with detoxification, antioxidant vitamins such as A, C and E is taken as well. Some individuals may feel that fasting would be the easiest route to detoxification. This may help, but anyone considering this route should discuss this with their healthcare provider, and if getting the go ahead, should be done under their supervision. Personal attention to products used, and caution in the use of these products, plus following the above health hints, can greatly improve one's health and strengthen the immune system.

POOR BIOENERGETICS

Conditioning is one of those areas of performance enhancement that is rarely calculated and precisely planned, as opposed to strength training. Granted, conditioning is very beneficial for overall health. After all, who doesn't want a stronger heart, efficient lungs, and overall health? Nonetheless, too much of a good thing can become detrimental, even with conditioning.

For starters, the body is not a machine. Its materials and tissues are subject to the same natural forces and laws of physics that all other known materials in the universe are subject to. This primarily includes fatigue and failure of materials that are repeatedly stressed. However, as discussed in the article "Understanding the Human Body - An Engineering Perspective", the body's feedback control system allows the materials to be repaired. Of course, time (i.e. rest) and resources (i.e. nutrition) are the factors governing recovery. Lack of monitoring and planning of aerobic volume and intensity can lead to premature over-training.

Far too often, athletes are pushed to their aerobic limits without a proper context for the workout session. Oftentimes, aerobically taxing workouts can be perceived to be more difficult by athletes and coaches as the activity can temporarily deprive the athlete of oxygen, inducing a state of hypoxia. This creates a very "tough" environment for the athlete and is measured by the ratings of perceived exertion scale. However, this type of practice can be detrimental to the performance of an athlete, depending on the exact sport.

It is crucial to realize that there is always a trade-off between endurance and power. Each time an athlete performs an activity, the nervous system takes into account the exact nature of the activity including its power output, and makes the necessary changes and adaptations to better cope with the induced stress. Just because the athlete did a session of weightlifting and then follows with an aerobic activity doesn't necessarily mean the athlete will derive the maximum benefits from each activity, when measured separately. Instead, both activities directly influence each other based on a power continuum. If not addressed, the athlete will only be "going in circles" with respect to maximal improvements for his/her sport.

When concerning athletic performance enhancement, the most interesting concept regarding endurance and strength training is the idea of this power continuum. Essentially, the laws of thermodynamics govern the power output that the body is capable of. An engine that is very powerful cannot also be very fuel-efficient. This is simply impossible since, by definition, power is the rate of energy production/consumption. Alternatively, a fuel-efficient engine cannot be equally powerful.

What implication does this have for athletic performance enhancement? Practically, an athlete cannot maximize his/her aerobic and power potential at the same point in time. Greater endurance is analogous to having more fuel-efficient muscles, while having more power is analogous to exactly that, more powerful muscles.

In addition, the sources of energy vary depending on the power output of the activity. When analyzed using thermodynamics, different types of fuels are capable of different rates of energy production. For instance, fossil fuels are a form of chemical energy, are highly reactive, and allow for faster generation of usable energy than say, electrical energy. In biological systems biochemical energy exists in the form of adenosine triphosphate, or ATP. Fast twitch fibers that require the shortest, yet highest bursts of power rely on stored energy in the form of creatine phosphate. Alternatively, slow twitch fibers involved with longer, lower power outputs rely on continuous energy generative processes such as glycolosis and ketosis, for instance. Usable ATP is generated from blood sugar as well as stored fat. Naturally, these processes are slower at generating energy than with creatine phosphate for fast movements.

Thus, when conditioning an athlete, some power characteristics may be sacrificed. As discussed in the article "Train what YOU can Train", the properties of muscle (e.g. fast twitch vs slow twitch) have not been shown to change to a large degree, if at all. In fact, changes for endurance athletes when compared to strength athletes consist mainly of biochemical changes with the aerobic enzymes and mitochondria, the power plant of the muscle cells. In addition, the number of capillaries, or the highways supplying the building blocks for energy, may increase with higher endurance activities.

Most importantly, motor recruitment strategies may be affected. The size principle has been hypothesized to explain how muscle fibers are normally recruited in untrained athletes. Those that are lower threshold (i.e. slow twitch) are recruited first, followed by higher threshold fibers (e.g. fast twitch), all in sequence. With training, the brain attempts to adapt to the stress levels of the activity and recruit muscles in the most efficient manner possible. Given the fact that strength training and endurance are on opposite ends of the power spectrum, combining both forms of training should cause some discrepancy in motor recruitment strategies, theoretically.

More specifically, heavy strength training requires the most energy consumption in the shortest period of time. Through repeated training sessions, the nervous system adapts by recruiting the higher threshold, larger, stronger fast-twitch fibers first. This is known as selective recruitment and is a strategy employed by the nervous system to maximize power output which consequently drains the muscle's stored ATP the fastest.

Alternatively, endurance training trains the nervous system to rely on mostly the slow twitch fibers. These fibers rely on slower energy mediums and aren't as adapted to high power but can generate moderate levels of power for extended periods. Thus, there is a training dilemma for the athletic performance specialist in terms of energy demands and bioenergetics.

In order to prepare the athlete fully for the endurance demands of his/her sport, an energy costs analysis must be performed. The major facets of this type of analysis include:

1. Estimating work (i.e. time performing activity) to rest ratio

2. Estimating average and maximal power outputs

In general, work to rest ratios will vary inversely with average power outputs. Specifically, higher work to rest ratios indicate higher endurance demands. For instance, a sport like football involves relatively longer periods of rest and higher maximal power outputs. When ranked by maximal power outputs, sports like baseball and football may be highest. Sports like basketball and soccer require higher endurance demands, but still have a power component.

Another way to visualize this continuum involves the cylinders of an engine. The ways in which the muscles of the athlete have been trained represent the engine. For instance, a V12 is analogous to a 100-m sprinter, high jumper, shot-putter, and weightlifter, to name a few. A V2 may be analogous to a marathon runner. A football wide-receiver may be a V10, while a basketball player may be a V8. A soccer player may be a V6. This is a gross analogy but provides a relative ranking and example of how energy costs demands vary with maximal power demands as observed in these sports.

Ultimately, how one trains for endurance is the key. There are various means to mimic the energy demands of the sport. Resistance training provides the stimulus for maximizing power output. Rest periods may be adjusted to train for more power endurance. If the sport is geared more towards power, then the endurance training can be incorporated into the framework of the strength training regimen. The length of the rest periods is based on the sport. On the other end of the spectrum, light loads (e.g. bodyweight) with low rest periods provide an environment for lower power outputs geared towards long-term endurance.

CHAPTER 4

RISK FACTORS 2

Congestive heart failure is one of the leading causes of death in the world and unless you ensure that you minimize the risk factors that bring on this problem, you could be at risk too. It is so important to try and prevent coronary disease by following a healthy lifestyle and letting your doctor guide you about how best to go about this.

Heart Attacks Happen

The arteries or the plumbing in your body through which the blood is carried to every part of your body, needs to be clear so that the oxygen-rich blood can flow and nourish every part. However, when the arteries get clogged due to sticky blood or plaque, they tend to get narrow and there could be the danger of blood clots blocking these narrow openings and causing angina or even a heart attack. This condition which is called atherosclerosis is the reason for most coronary heart disease problems. This can be prevented by following a healthy lifestyle and eliminating the risk factors that lead to this problem.

Most Common Risk Factors

There are certain risk factors that make you prone to coronary diseases and by ensuring that you take them out of your life, you could prevent or minimize the possibility of attacks.

• Cigarettes: Smoking is one of the main culprits and nicotine not only thickens the blood and makes it sticky, it also deprives it of oxygen. When the blood gets thicker, it moves more sluggishly and it can cause plaque and blockages.

• Cholesterol and BP levels: If your 'bad' cholesterol or LDL levels are high or if your Blood Pressure is over the normal levels, you could run the risk of coronary problems so it would be wise to keep these under control with healthy eating, exercise and medication.

• Obesity and Lack of Exercise: Both factors run the risk of pressure on the heart and you need to change your lifestyle habits, factor in regular exercise and make an effort to lose weight.

• History of Heart Disease: If you are genetically prone to coronary disease, all the more reason to ensure that you take preventive action and do everything you can to follow a healthy lifestyle and prevent getting a heart attack.

• Diabetes: If you are a diabetic, make sure you keep your sugar levels under control and exercise regularly so you ease the pressure on your heart.

• Depression: This needs to be treated because it is one of the risk factors of heart disease.

GENETIC

In the last decade, studies in men and women have shown that inflammation is an important risk factor for heart disease, perhaps equal in importance to unhealthy cholesterol levels. Recent scientific discoveries indicate that some of the risk for cardiovascular disease, including heart attacks, is due to variations in the genes that we inherit. Just as with conventional cardiovascular risk factors such as high cholesterol, smoking and diabetes, the presence of one or more of these DNA variations does not mean that an individual will develop cardiovascular disease. However, using knowledge about genetic risk factors to make informed choices about diet and lifestyle may reduce your risk of developing cardiovascular disease in the future.

Gensona Heart Health is the first and only genetic test that analyzes two interleukin 1 (IL1) genes for variations that identify an individual's predisposition for over-expression of inflammation and risk for cardiovascular disease. IL1 genetic susceptibility may not initiate or cause heart disease but rather may lead to earlier or more severe disease. This test is not intended to and does not diagnose a specific disease. The IL1 genetic test can be used to differentiate certain IL1 genotypes associated with varying inflammatory responses to identify individuals at risk for cardiovascular disease and heart attacks even before age 60.

The IL1 genetic test for heart health is based on scientific data from genetic association studies obtained through research collaborations with scientific experts in cardiovascular disease at leading academic institutions. This exclusive, patented test developed by Interleukin uses the latest medical research and technology to provide the best available genetic information to help make decisions aimed at preserving heart health.

The genetic test provides risk information independent of traditional risk factors (such as family history, hypertension and smoking) in assessing risk for heart disease. The IL1 composite genotypes are as important as many of the standard risk factors currently associated with heart disease. A positive result means that the DNA pattern in your IL1 genes is associated with a tendency to increased inflammation and to heart disease before you reach the age of 60. Individuals who test positive have about twice the risk of heart attacks when compared with individuals who are at the lowest level of risk.

Knowledge of an individual's IL1 genotype identifies a life-long influence on inflammation, which can be modulated by preventive actions. The IL1 composite genotypes associated with increased risk are common in most ethnic and racial groups. Knowing predisposition to inflammation can help one to develop a personalized health plan (nutrition and lifestyle) for risk reduction. Nutritional and lifestyle decisions targeting the reduction of inflammation induced by IL1 may improve heart health.

EMOTIONAL STRESS

There is no doubt that a common cause of heart disease is stress. Stress and heart disease have been associated with each other for years. It is important to learn to recognize stress and take appropriate steps to avoid all the harmful effects. Plenty of research has been conducted on the relation between stress and how it can lead to heart troubles. Stress can also lead to many people developing coronary problems at a very early age.

Stress is known to be among the number one killers, especially with the busy lifestyles that many people live. Added pressures at work and on the domestic front only exacerbate the problem further.

Stress typically leads to high blood pressure, which in turn leads to heart disease. Stress also increases the cholesterol levels in the body, which is once again a major cause for a heart condition. Overeating can be a result of stress, leading to weight gain and consequently to heart problems. Other bad habits such as smoking and drinking are also associated with stress, while smoking is known to be a cause for heart disease. Hence, directly or indirectly, stress seems to be linked to heart disease in many ways.

Prolonged periods of stress can lead to a weak immune system. This in turn lowers the body's resistance to illnesses and weakens the heart as well. With such compelling evidence, there is no doubt that stress and heart disease are related. If stress can be controlled it can be the first step towards preventing heart disease.

Most people undergo plenty of job stress that can have a negative impact on their health, especially the cardiovascular system. There have been several studies conducted on the relation between job stress and heart disease. Researchers have undertaken the study of individuals who have returned to the job place after experiencing a heart attack. According to observations in the first six weeks and once again two years later, people who returned to a stressful job were more likely to experience another heart attack as compared to those with stress free jobs.

There is good stress as well as bad stress that exists. Good stress can be emotional or physical and is generally experienced in short bursts. Physical stress includes activities such as exercise which is good for the heart. Emotional stress can be experienced when you try something new or face a sudden fearful situation that does not last long. Bad stress on the other hand is prolonged and low lever stress where the body is exposed to high levels of cortisol or 'stress hormone' which is released by the body, thereby increasing the risk of coronary disease.

The bottom line to beat stress and heart disease is to lead a healthy lifestyle, stick to a diet, exercise regularly, and learn to cope with situations in a better manner so that stress does not get the better of you.

CHAPTER 5

You live a very comfortable life. You party until the wee hours of the morning. You smoke like there is no tomorrow. You guzzle liquor like water. You never exercise or exert any kind of effort, because you do not like the feel of sweat rolling down your forehead. And after years of this lifestyle, time seems to have taken its toll.

At the present time, you are experiencing some chest pains, coupled with shortness of breath each time you try to walk some distance. You never thought that this would happen to you, even with the kind of lifestyle you lead. But now you realize that you are not as omnipotent and mighty as you thought you were.

One of your friends refers you to a doctor. The doctor is not just any kind of doctor. Your friend has referred you to a doctor who specializes in heart problems - a cardiologist.

Generally, cardiology is a branch of medicine. And just like any other branch, cardiology has a specific function and focus. It has anything and everything to do with the heart and its specific functions. Cardiology covers disorders of the heart, disorders of the blood vessels, diagnosis and cures for diseases and malfunctions of this vital organ.

At some point in there life, virtually everyone will experience severe chest pain. This is because chest pain can have a number of causes including indigestion and something even as simple as a stressed or pulled muscle in the back. However; there are cases where severe chest pain can be a symptom of heart disease. Heart disease can strike at any time in a persons life and afflicts both men and women.

Nine Million Americans At Risk

At the present time over nine-million Americans are at immediate risk of heart disease and the vast majority of them don't even know it. However; in recent decades great strides have been made in understanding and detecting this silent killer but the first step that must be taken is to undergo a cardiology test and report.

Myocardial Profusion Imaging

One common type of heart disease is known as coronary artery disease or CAD, which is when the arteries surrounding and connecting to the heart become clogged or impeded. One of the most common tests for detecting and gaging the severity of this type pf coronary artery blockage is called Myocardial Perfusion Imaging.

Nuclear Camera

To perform this test, a benign fluid that contains a mildly radioactive substance is injected into the person receiving the test. Then a nuclear camera is used to obtain three dimensional images of the actual blood flow in the arteries in and around the heart. The camera can't detect the blood itself but it can see the mildly radioactive material that is in the blood, so the cardiologist is able to get an actual inside view of the arteries that my be obstructed.

A Course of Treatment

After the test is completed, a complete report is then written up detailing the results of the test. With this report a physician can then determine and prescribe a course of treatment that can include medication and exercise or surgery. Without the test, and subsequent report however, arterial blockage of the coronary arteries can be and often is fatal.

For cardiologists to find out what condition your heart is in, they perform a complete physical check up and examination first. The results provide data regarding your heart's condition. Along with that, you will be asked about your health history and your family's as well. You will also be asked about your lifestyle and habits. This may seem totally unrelated to your condition, however these pieces of information will give the cardiologist answers regarding your heart condition.

Cardiology also entails several examinations, tests and procedures for patients complaining about possible heart problems. These could include an ultrasound of your heart, a cardiac stress test, an electrocardiogram (or also known as ECG and EKG) and the use of a blood pressure cuff among many others.

Is a Heart Scan the Right Test For You?

We have heard the stories about a friend who visits his doctor and has a clean bill of health. Two days later he dies of a massive heart attack and you do not understand how or why this happened. Your friend was active, played handball regularly, he was thin, and he ate fish. His total cholesterol was a little high but his good cholesterol was very good. He was taking a low dose of medication to keep his blood pressure down for about a year and that was working. What happened?

Blood pressure and cholesterol levels are reliable gauges of how much at risk you are for heart disease. However, the amount of calcium in your coronary arteries and how it is affecting your blood flow may be an even better way of predicting who is most likely to have a heart attack unless they get on medication therapy.

The problem is that someone who is asymptomatic, in good shape, active and eats well is not sending any red flares that something is wrong. Without any symptoms such as shortness of breath or high blood pressure even with medication, there is no indication that he needs a heart scan, also known as Coronary Calcium Scans.

Heart scans use noninvasive techniques that measure the amount of calcium in the walls of your coronary arteries, the arteries that supply your heart with blood. One of the goals of cardiac CT for calcium scoring is to determine if coronary artery disease, CAD, is present and to what extent, even if there are no symptoms. It is a screening for patients with risk factors for CAD but no clinical symptoms because having calcium in the walls of your arteries could mean you have coronary artery disease, a major cause of heart attacks. CAD takes place when plaque builds up and narrows your arteries.

The plaques are made of fat, cholesterol and calcium. It is the calcium in those plaques that the CT scan detects. The CT scan obtains information about the presence, location and extent of calcified plaque in the coronary arteries. The amount of calcium that is present is used to calculate a score that, when combined with your other health information, helps to determine your risk of coronary heart disease or heart attack. The result of this test is called a coronary calcium score.

However, heart scans are still controversial. First they are not for everyone.

What' is more, it is still unclear whether heart scans should be used widely. Routine use of heart scans on people who do not have any symptoms of heart disease is also not recommended by the American Heart Association or the American College of Cardiology.

They report that a heart scan is not useful if you have a low heart attack risk. For example, if you are younger than 55 years old, have normal cholesterol and blood pressure levels and do no't smoke, your heart attack risk is less than 10 percent and a heart scan is not going to tell your doctor something he does not already know. On the other hand if you are at high risk because you are over 65, your cholesterol is high and so is your blood pressure, the heart scan may not do you much good either because you and your doctor already know you are at high risk.

If on the other hand, you fall somewhere between the two and have borderline high cholesterol or high blood pressure you may find having a heart scan will give you valuable information. You will be able to tell more precisely what your risk of CAD is.

The theory behind using heart scans is that the more calcification you have, the worse your heart disease. Part of the theory is that even having small amounts of calcium might indicate you could go on to develop heart disease unless you take aggressive measures to stop it such as reducing your cholesterol and living a more healthy lifestyle.

However, having calcium in your coronary arteries does not mean you have heart disease. How much do you pay attention to the dreaded false-positive results? That means there is an error on the scan. For instance, if you show heart disease your doctor may request more invasive tests that would not be necessary because there was a mistake.

On the other hand, the heart scan can show you are free of calcium and that does not mean you absolutely do not have heart disease. The plaques that build up in your arteries start out as soft and only become calcified over time. So your arteries can be clogged but the scan cannot detect them.

CHAPTER 6

MEDICATION TO TREAT HEART DISEASE

Heart disease is a general term for a number of different diseases, all of which influence the heart in some way. Heart disease is in fact considered as being the leading reason of death nowadays in the United States. Heart disease indeed possesses serious threat to many people. Therefore, it is important to understand the methods to prevent and treat heart disease.

Prevention methods

There is reason to be hopeful because according to experts, heart disease prevention is promising. Even though some risk factors including sex, genetics, and age of a person are not within our control, one can still make an alteration in lifestyle and also change diet so that the odds of heart disease are significantly reduced.

There are also other methods by which heart disease prevention can be achieved. According to what the American Heart Association proposes, one must control obesity even in children and also make a determined attempt to take proper diet that contains enough nutrition. One of the better nutritional supplements you may want to try for heart disease prevention is mangosteen puree that is rich in antioxidants which aid in destroying free radicals that are the reason behind damage to cells and which in turn will result in heart disease.

Good heart disease prevention may also mean controlling the blood pressure and having LDL cholesterol at low levels. The best way to attain these goals is by making appropriate changes to diet and even by taking medications if so recommended by the doctor. Clearly, having low blood sugar levels will consider as heart disease prevention.

Another alternative is to exercise because it is a well known fact that regular exercise can reduce the risks of heart disease. Experts have a tendency to recommend as much exercise as humanly possible at least an hour per day. For many people, this seems like a never-ending task but the truth is this amount of exercise can be attained in ways other than going to the gym. Basically changing some habits, such as walking to work, can make people healthier. Walking is perhaps the easiest, cheapest, and healthiest type of exercise for most people and therefore should be taken advantage of.

The best heart disease prevention may not be a solitary course of action; rather, one may decide to have many strategies combined into one that will prove to be more effective. You can select approaches such as changes in diet, together with reducing excess weight and also maintaining blood sugar levels as well as taking nutritional supplements that are suggested by health experts.

Treatment options for heart disease

If you have heart disease then you will have to have some types of heart disease treatment in order to solve your problem. There are various heart disease treatment options that are available nowadays. The first treatment is of course prevention as explained previously.

However, if your heart disease is serious, than most probably you will also have to use more serious techniques of heart disease treatment. This includes medical treatment, which will usually be started straight away, even before an exact diagnosis of a heart problem is made.

This medical treatment may comprise of oxygen from a tube in the nose, oxygen through a face mask, nitroglycerin under the tongue, pain medicines, and aspirin. There are also clot dissolving medications which are often given, and the earlier these drugs are given, the higher the chances of opening the blocked artery and defending the cardiac muscle from further injury.

Cellular therapy, for example, is considered as being a potential treatment for heart disease. This is due to cellular products have been revealed to hold great potential for the treating of injured and diseased tissues in the body. They come from many sources, such as stem cells from bone marrow, peripheral blood, and myoblasts from skeletal muscle cells. The research so far has shown that this cellular therapy offers amazingly positive results, and so with additional research and more advancement, in the future this just may be known as the cure for heart disease.

Surgery can be executed on those who experience heart disease at any age although other methods are preferable. Surgery is necessary for those who do not react to their medications or whose condition worsens radically. In some situations, surgery is the only method to amend the problem and give the patient a probability of good health. In uncommon cases, repeat surgery is needed afterward to rid the body of excess fluids that have developed in the chest.

Heart surgery can be wearing and the healing period can be slow so it is no surprise to find out that a huge number of people who suffer from heart disease which needs surgery are interested in less invasive surgery. Less invasive surgery for heart disease can involve smaller incisions, less pain, and a much faster healing period. Not only does this type of surgery involve shorter hospital stays, it can also reduce the risks of complications to the patient during and after the operation.

There are many resources that are available if you want more information on the treatment of heart disease. The most significant thing of all is to keep a healthy lifestyle, a healthy and nutritious diet, and plenty of exercise. By keeping a healthy lifestyle you will not only be guarding yourself against heart disease but as well against all illnesses and health conditions in general.

Medications used for treating heart disease include beta blockers. These medications slow and strengthen the contractions of the heart muscle so that it does not have to work hard. In addition, beta blockers are very effective in treating pain from angina, or chest pain. Although they can cause significant side effects such as fatigue, dizziness, weakness and cold extremities, beta blockers can greatly increase cardiac output and might even prevent a heart attack.

A heart healthy diet, or a diet that is low in fat is also effective in treating heart disease. It is best for patients who are already dealing with the disease to receive nutritional counseling and support from a professional nutritionist. A healthy diet that is low fat, but that also adds the necessary nutrients for a healthy body, can be customized for each patient. The follow-up to a healthy diet plan is to add a safe, healthy exercise routine to a patient's weekly schedule. While over-exercising can be a danger, the right amount of moderate exercise under to supervision of a physician, can strengthen the heart and often add longevity to one's lifespan.

A healthy diet and moderate exercise also promotes weight loss and lower blood pressure, which are both risk factors in the development of heart disease. Eating a diet that is nutritionally healthy and participating in an appropriate fitness program can not only help to avoid the effects of heart disease, but it also can help other conditions as well. It is important however, to speak to a health care professional before starting an exercise routine, especially when established heart disease is already present.

Treating Heart Disease With Aspirin

The practice of prescribing aspirin to patients with heart disease goes back to the 1940s, but it took a long time before studies proved what general practitioners had noticed. Aspirin can prevent blood clots and reduce the risk of heart attacks. This was finally proved to everyone's satisfaction in 1989.

Aspirin has been around a long time, and even before it was made into a pill, it was used in its natural form. Willow bark contains the same ingredient and is how the first aspirin tablets were made.

As mentioned in the teaser, aspirin has both pros and cons. Most of the time, the good it does outweighs the bad, but knowing them could save your life.

Pros

Pain Killer: Headaches, muscle strains and other types of pain can be relieved with this product. It can be helpful both by swallowing it and by putting it on the skin. There are over the counter creams and gels that help you stop the pain topically.

Fevers: While it is not as strong as some other products, aspirin (and before that willow) has been used to treat all kinds of fevers. It doesn't matter what the cause, it works across the board.

Blood Thinner: Unlike other NSAIDs, aspirin can thin the blood enough to prevent heart attacks. Some doctors recommend starting an aspirin regimen even for those who don't have any of the symptoms of the problem, just as a preventative measure.

Cons

Allergies: There are a number of people who are allergic to aspirin. Taking it can cause breathing problems sometimes severe enough to kill. If you notice any changes to your breathing, a feeling of being chocked or any other respiratory problem, call your doctor. You may need a trip to the emergency room.

Bleeding in the Digestive Tract: The chemical in this product causes small cuts to the digestive tract. You may notice a change in your stools after taking it. Tell your doctor if you find this, as you may need to reduce the dose.

Clotting Disorders: Because it is a blood thinner, those with clotting disorders should avoid aspirin unless prescribed by a doctor that is aware of your condition. It could make the disorder worse.

Gout: Aspirin is a direct cause of gout flareups. The higher the dosage, the more at risk you are. Be sure to discuss this with your doctor if it is prescribed for you. The last thing you need is this extremely painful disorder on top of dealing with a life threatening medical condition.

Upset Stomach: Despite the buffering agent, this product can upset your stomach. Be sure to take it with food in order to prevent that side effect. If the problem continues, your doctor may want to change the dosage or prescribe a medication to block that effect.

It's not a good idea to self diagnose or self prescribe. It's also unwise to stop taking a medication prescribed by your doctor without discussing it. To protect yourself, make an appointment and find out if aspirin therapy will benefit you.

CHAPTER 7

DETOX

Body detox is among the best ways of keeping ourselves clean and healthy, besides other methods such as special diets, vitamin supplements, natural therapies, and so on. An important step in a full body detox is to restore or also to replenish energy levels to make you more alert in different areas of your life, such as at work. A body cleanse or body detox is also a great way to give your body a boost after a night of over-indulgence, eating all the wrong foods and consuming more alcohol than is healthy. That is why body detox is needed because some mortals are having this kind of lifestyle.

The human body has a built in detox system that removes harmful substances from the body through excretion but when we put pressure on it by eating unhealthy foods, drinking too much alcohol and not getting enough sleep the system is weakened. At one time, the need for a natural body detox seemed to apply only to those who suffered from some form of drug or alcohol dependency. The pollution your body is exposed to daily, and your consumption of various types of junk food, coffee, aerated drinks, alcohol etc leads to the accumulation of various toxins in your body. Initially known for elimination of excessive alcohol and drugs from the body, detox is now being used more extensively for the process of elimination of any kind of toxins that may be present in the body. A full body detox diet plan using raw vegetables and fresh fruits is especially recommended for young individuals whose bodies have been subjected to high levels of alcohol, burgers and pizzas.

Today's refined diets, stressful lifestyles antibiotics or other health problems can deplete the body's natural store of these little miracle workers and upset the delicate balance or eubiosis. There are numerous other methods to detox your body, such as through herbal tea and supplements, in addition to specialized diets and spa programs. Body detox diets vary but typically involve eating or drinking nothing but raw, steamed or gently stir-fried vegetables and fruit, pulses, sprouted seeds, thin soups, juices and plain cereals such as brown rice, millet or buckwheat. Mediterranean diets are low on fat and carbohydrates and they provide us with healthy alternative to the oily food we consume every day.

Start using the benefit of exercise to cleanse and detoxify your body. Exercise increases oxygen to your system and raises your body temperature, in effect combining oxygen therapy and hyperthermia. Exercise detoxification is an effective method of cleansing many vital organs simultaneously and should become a regular part of your life. There are tons of exercise programs and plans out there, or just walking for at least 12-15 minutes a day is beneficial to the colon function. The simplest form of administering oxygen therapy is through a simple deep breathing exercise.

The increase in the amount of toxins in the body results in stress in the immune system that eventually breaks down due to overwork. If you are interested in the idea of detoxing and want to receive the fastest results possible, then what you are going to want to do is find a quick detox diet, a body detox that is going to offer you quick results. Some methods are used individually as body detox solutions while other individuals use several methods together to achieve the best possible results. If you want to receive optimum results from your detox, you should consider taking some supplements for detox. It is also good for keeping track of detox intervals or a detox schedule, body detox is not just a one time thing, for best results it should be done on a regular basis throughout the year.

While our body is not totally defenseless against toxins as we have an effective built-in natural detoxification system but body detox is still a must to help keep your body free of toxins. One of the much-desired benefits of body detox is weight loss. Liver and Kidneys detox is excellent to use before and during a weight loss program, as it will improve weight loss results. In conclusion, making your own home remedy for body detox is much better and less expensive way to pursue long term health as compared to eating detox pills.

Body detox is among the best ways of keeping ourselves clean and healthy, besides other methods such as special diets, vitamin supplements, natural therapies, and so on. An important step in a full body detox is to restore or also to replenish energy levels to make you more alert in different areas of your life, such as at work. A body cleanse or body detox is also a great way to give your body a boost after a night of over-indulgence, eating all the wrong foods and consuming more alcohol than is healthy. That is why body detox is needed because some mortals are having this kind of lifestyle.

The human body has a built in detox system that removes harmful substances from the body through excretion but when we put pressure on it by eating unhealthy foods, drinking too much alcohol and not getting enough sleep the system is weakened. At one time, the need for a natural body detox seemed to apply only to those who suffered from some form of drug or alcohol dependency. The pollution your body is exposed to daily, and your consumption of various types of junk food, coffee, aerated drinks, alcohol etc leads to the accumulation of various toxins in your body. Initially known for elimination of excessive alcohol and drugs from the body, detox is now being used more extensively for the process of elimination of any kind of toxins that may be present in the body. A full body detox diet plan using raw vegetables and fresh fruits is especially recommended for young individuals whose bodies have been subjected to high levels of alcohol, burgers and pizzas.

Today's refined diets, stressful lifestyles antibiotics or other health problems can deplete the body's natural store of these little miracle workers and upset the delicate balance or eubiosis. There are numerous other methods to detox your body, such as through herbal tea and supplements, in addition to specialized diets and spa programs. Body detox diets vary but typically involve eating or drinking nothing but raw, steamed or gently stir-fried vegetables and fruit, pulses, sprouted seeds, thin soups, juices and plain cereals such as brown rice, millet or buckwheat. Mediterranean diets are low on fat and carbohydrates and they provide us with healthy alternative to the oily food we consume every day.

Start using the benefit of exercise to cleanse and detoxify your body. Exercise increases oxygen to your system and raises your body temperature, in effect combining oxygen therapy and hyperthermia. Exercise detoxification is an effective method of cleansing many vital organs simultaneously and should become a regular part of your life. There are tons of exercise programs and plans out there, or just walking for at least 12-15 minutes a day is beneficial to the colon function. The simplest form of administering oxygen therapy is through a simple deep breathing exercise.

The increase in the amount of toxins in the body results in stress in the immune system that eventually breaks down due to overwork. If you are interested in the idea of detoxing and want to receive the fastest results possible, then what you are going to want to do is find a quick detox diet, a body detox that is going to offer you quick results. Some methods are used individually as body detox solutions while other individuals use several methods together to achieve the best possible results. If you want to receive optimum results from your detox, you should consider taking some supplements for detox. It is also good for keeping track of detox intervals or a detox schedule, body detox is not just a one time thing, for best results it should be done on a regular basis throughout the year.

While our body is not totally defenseless against toxins as we have an effective built-in natural detoxification system but body detox is still a must to help keep your body free of toxins. One of the much-desired benefits of body detox is weight loss. Liver and Kidneys detox is excellent to use before and during a weight loss program, as it will improve weight loss results. In conclusion, making your own home remedy for body detox is much better and less expensive way to pursue long term health as compared to eating detox pills.

CONCLUSION

Heart disease is the #1 killer in the United States today. This may not be a surprise to many of you. What may surprise you is that a heart attack is avoidable in many cases. Unfortunately heart defects do not fall into this category and can not be prevented but you can take actions to prevent much of the heart disease that causes heart attacks.

Through quick response and education most heart attacks are not fatal. 75% of men and 60% of women survive and continue living at least a year. Still it has been reported that 150,000 people die each year of heart attacks.

Heart attacks occur more frequently in the morning hours. This is because the blood platelets are especially sticky and more prone to clots. The average age of heart attack victims is 66 for men and 70 for women. The risk increases for men after the age of 45 and for women after the age of 55. Now I don't want all the women reading this report to wave it in the face of their favorite man quite yet because men that survive a heart attack usually live longer than women that survive an attack.

Enough of the gruesome facts, let's get on to how it is our choice. What can we do to prevent missing lunch or worse, the rest of our lives? There are three things within our control that play a big part in the likelihood of suffering a heart attack.

- Weight
- Diet
- Fitness

Control your weight.

It has been a long known fact that obesity increases a person's risk of heart disease. Something that has just recently been discovered is that waist size plays a bigger role in a person's risk than BMI (body mass index). Lopez-Jimenez and his colleagues from the Mayo Clinic tested nearly 16,000 heart patients who participated in one of four previously conducted studies. More than one-third of the patients died during the studies, which ranged in length from six months to more than seven years. They found that people with a high BMI had a 35% greater chance of survival than those with a larger waist size. When a high BMI was coupled with a large waist the chance of survival was cut in half. So, what's the choice? Decrease your waist size or increase your risk of heart attack.

Control your diet

Both quality and quantity of the foods you consume are vital in keeping your arteries fit and functioning. The quality of your consumption will keep your arteries clean and let blood flow smoothly. When you eat too many foods that are too high in saturated fats you increase your risk of building up cholesterol plaque. Most of us are aware that we have two kinds of cholesterol the "good", HDL, and the "bad", LDL. Let me help you understand the difference.. To put it as simply as I can, LDL is considered bad because it carries the cholesterol to the cell and if it carries to much, or more than the cell can use the LDL just hangs around and builds up into plaque. HDL gets the good reputation because it carries the cholesterol away from the cell back to the liver to be broken down or eliminated from the body as waste. So, what's the choice? Increase your HDL and decrease your LDL or increase your risk of heart attack.

Control your fitness

Your heart is just like any other muscle in your body. If you don't use it you lose it. You have heard it time and time again. All it takes is 30 minutes of aerobic exercise 3 to 4 times a week. With obesity and heart attack stealing our lives at an amazing rate it is time to fight back. Get that heart pumping. Aerobic exercise does not mean running marathons. It does not mean fitness club fees. You could drastically reduce your risk of heart attack and heart disease simply by taking a brisk walk around your neighborhood 3 or 4 times a week. If you don't currently get much exercise you should start slowly and work yourself up to walking a mile and a half in 30 to 35 minutes. Of course you want to check with your Dr. before making any changes to your diet or fitness program. You have your car checked for road worthy before any long trip, don't you? So what's the choice? Increase your heart rate three to four times a week or increase your risk of heart attack.

So you see, the choice truly is yours. When you take control of your weight, your diet and your fitness, you take control of your life.

THANK YOU FOR READING !